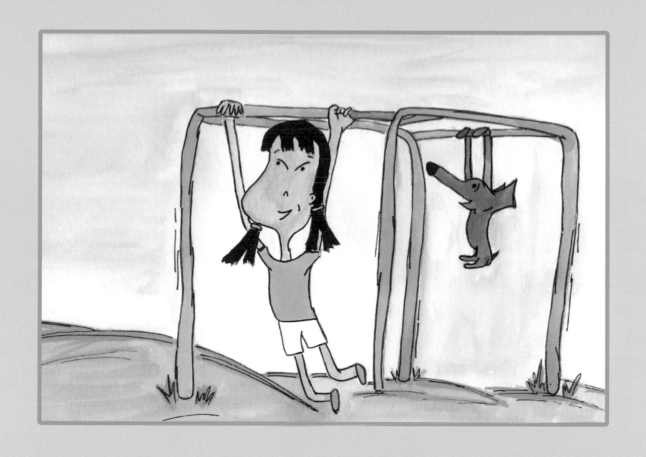

Meet Mei. Mei is courageous, active, and loves to play at the playground. Her favorite part is the monkey bars and the way she swings from bar to bar –
just like a monkey swings from vine to vine!

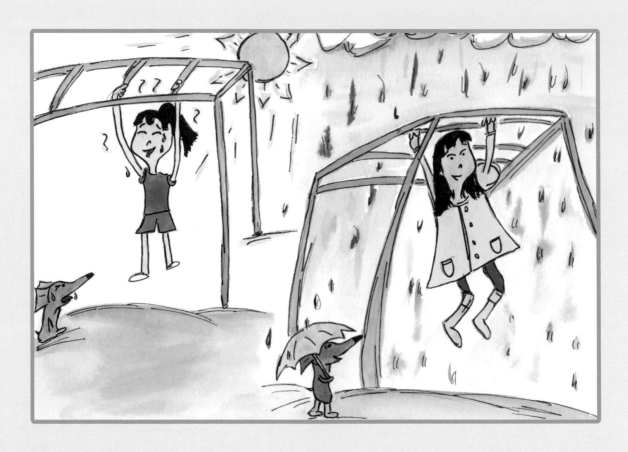

Mei goes to the monkey bars every day, regardless of the weather. It could be hot and steamy or raining cats and dogs. You'll find Mei there after school, every afternoon.

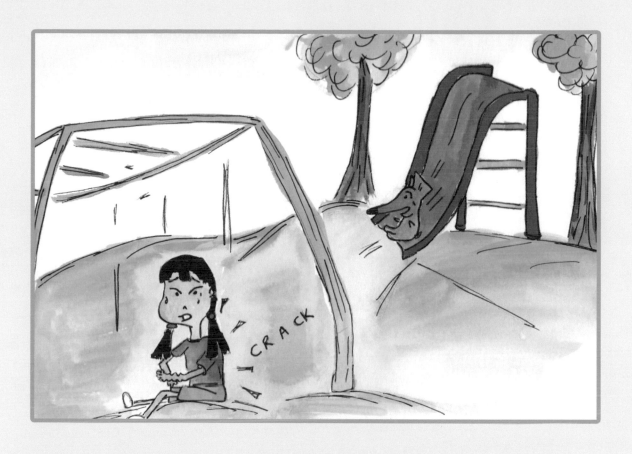

One day, after a thunderstorm had rolled through, Mei was happily swinging up and down the bars, singing to herself. All of a sudden, she felt her hands slip, as the bars were wet and slick from the rain. She fell down to the ground, landing smack dab on her arm with a loud CRACK!

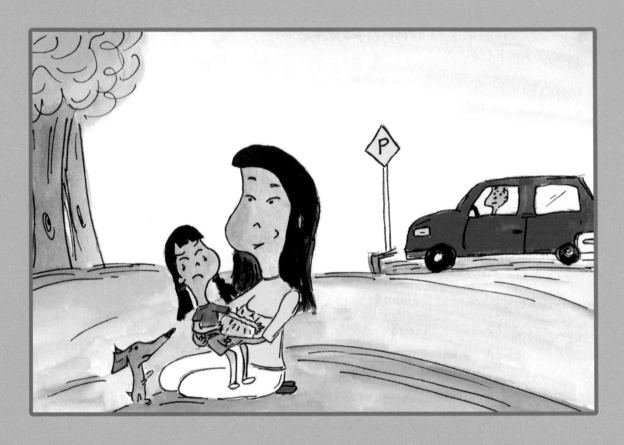

Mei felt pain racing up and down her arm. Tears sprang to her eyes. What had just happened? Her mom immediately scooped her up and off to the emergency department they went.

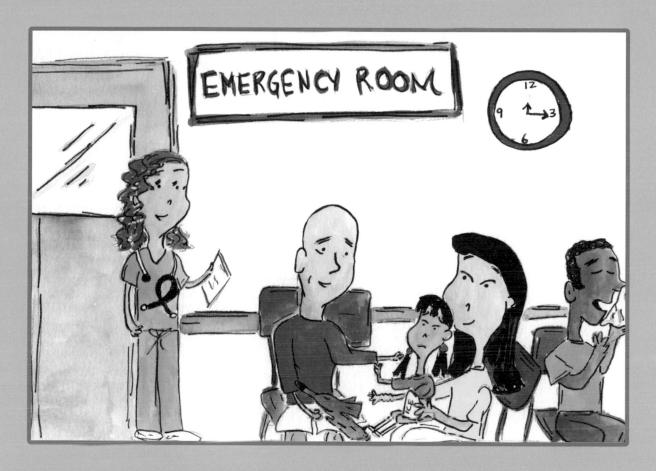

The emergency department was a busy and bustling place. There were all sorts of people there. Some were sneezing, some looked tired, and some were also holding their arms in pain. Mei tried to be brave as she patiently waited for her turn. Her mom put an ice pack on her arm to help with the pain – nice and cold!

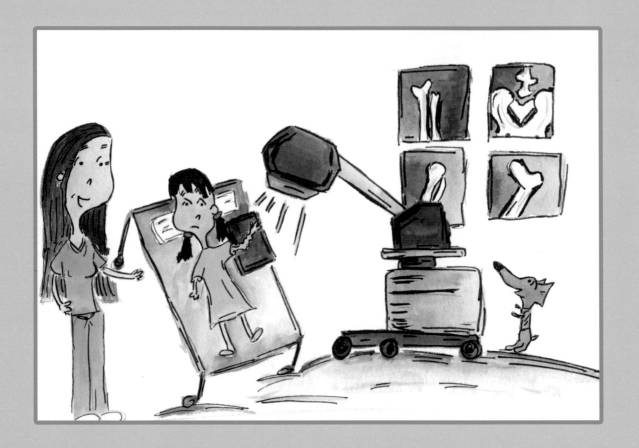

Then it was Mei's turn! First, pictures called x-rays were taken of her arm to look at her bones. These pictures showed that a bone in her arm was broken. It was called the radius and there was a crack running right through it – just like a lightning bolt!

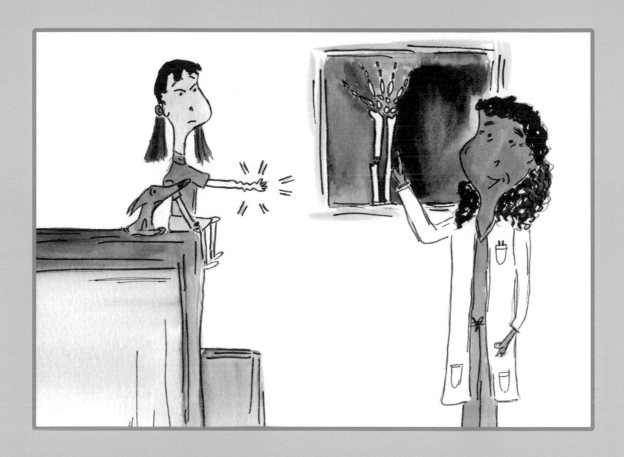

Mei had a broken arm! The doctor said she would need a cast and the monkey bars would be off limits until her bone healed. This is because broken bones need lots of rest to get better. But there was good news too — Mei could pick the color of her cast! She chose light blue with sparkles.

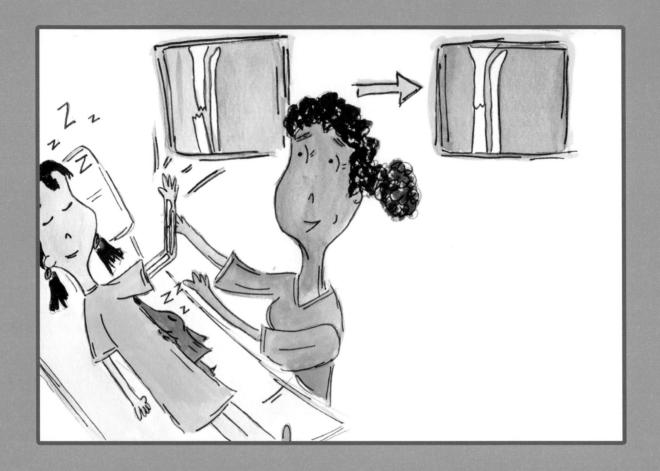

Mei's mommy and daddy held her hand while the doctor gave her medicine to make her very sleepy. She drifted off into dreamland filled with big, fluffy dogs. While she was sleeping, the doctor used an x-ray machine, and guided her bone back into the right place.

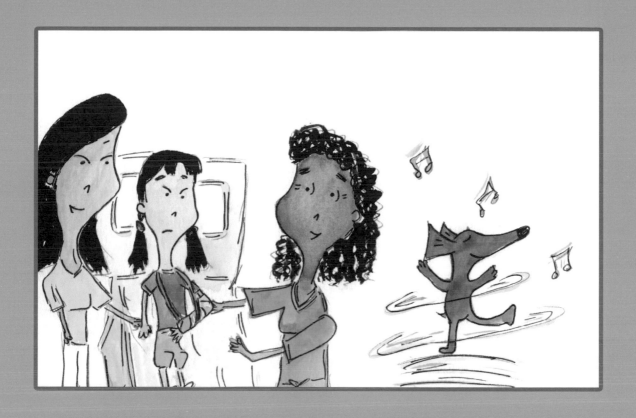

Mei's arm was wrapped with soft cotton very carefully.
Then a wet layer was added that hardened—like a shell—
to protect Mei's arm. This was her new cast! Next, her arm
was rested carefully in a sling, which was like a hammock
for her cast. The cast was to stay on for weeks.
What would she do without the monkey bars?

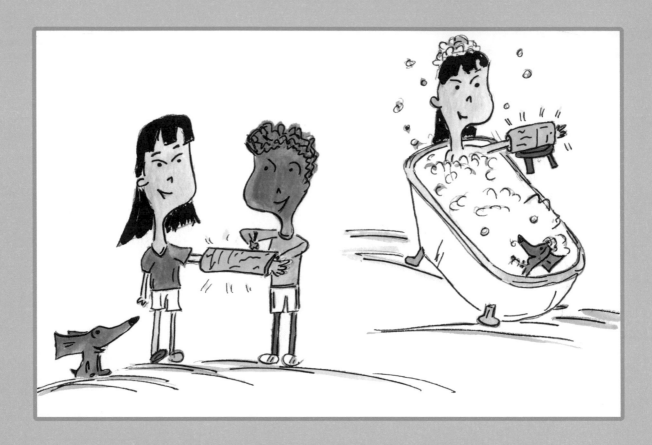

Over the next few weeks, Mei became a pro with her cast. Her family and friends signed it, making it even more colorful and special. She made sure to keep her cast dry, always covering it when she took a bath. And even when her arm itched, she didn't stick anything into the cast to scratch it. Good job, Mei!

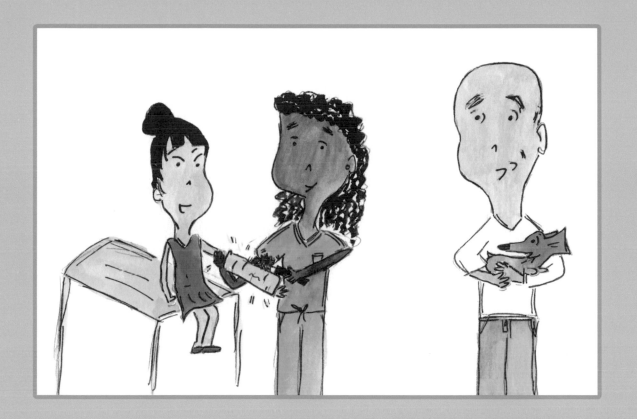

Before Mei knew it, it was time for the cast to be removed!
She went back to see the doctor and a special tool was used
to remove it. It looked like a saw but it wasn't sharp at all.
It just vibrated very loudly until the cast cracked open.

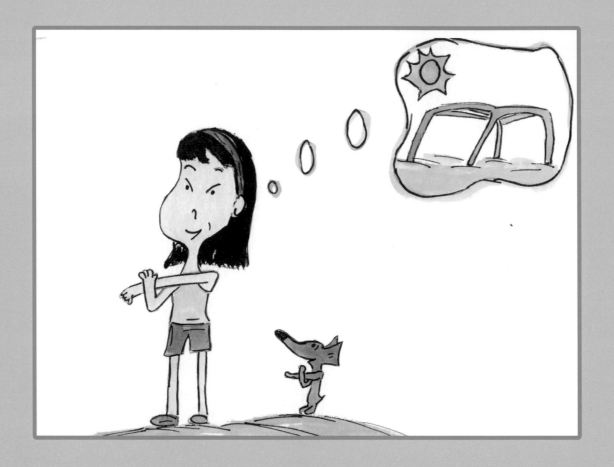

Mei's arm emerged, like a butterfly from its cocoon. Except, it looked paler and smaller than her other arm. Did it really belong to her? Her doctor showed her exercises to make her arm strong again so she could get back to the monkey bars. Mei did her exercises and every day her arm got stronger and stronger.

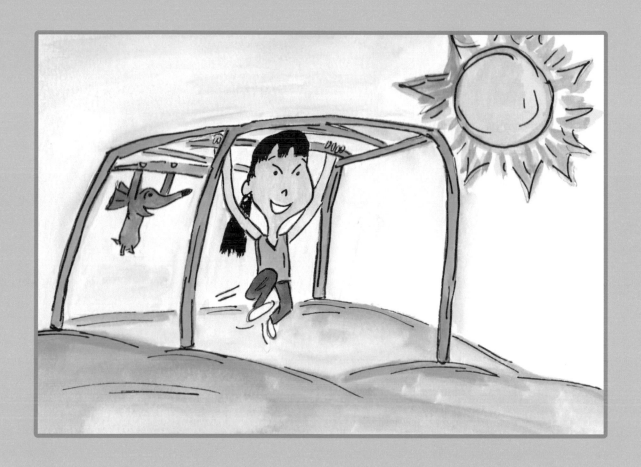

Until finally the time came, when Mei felt ready to face the monkey bars again. She showed up at the playground and slowly walked to the jungle gym. Climbing the ladder, she closed her eyes for a moment and then, without hesitation, grabbed the first monkey bar and started swinging excitedly! Mei was back!

Bone Facts

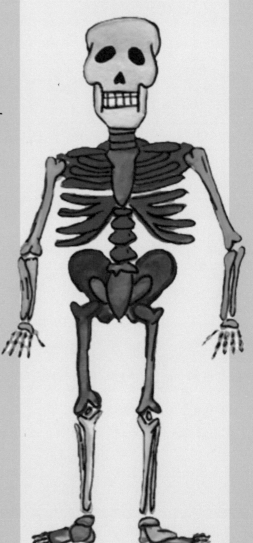

This colorful skeleton shows the many bones in your body!

1. When you are born, you have almost 300 bones in your body. Some of these bones fuse together until you have a total of 206 bones as a fully-grown adult.

2. Your bones are very important. They support your entire body and maintain your body's shape.

3. Bones let your body move and protect your insides.

4. Bones also produce blood cells and store minerals.

5. The smallest bone in your body is in your ear (stapes) and the longest bone is in your leg (femur).

6. Bones are strong and tough. They support you for your whole life! Of course, they can break (Mei knows that first-hand), but it takes a lot of force to break them.

7. To keep your bones strong, don't forget to exercise and eat healthy foods that contain calcium.

Fracture Facts

1. Broken bones, or fractures, are very common in kids because their bones are still growing. Therefore, they are more fragile and flexible then adult bones; however, this also means that they heal faster!

2. Up to 40% of girls and 50% of boys will have a fracture in childhood.

3. The most common causes of fractures are from accidents involving:
   a. Monkey bars
   b. Trampolines
   c. Scooters
   d. Snowboarding
   e. Sports

4. Fractures can happen anywhere in the body, but the most common locations in kids are wrists, arms, and elbows.

5. Signs of a fracture include pain, swelling, redness, and an unusual shape (deformity).

6. You can use an ice pack and elevate your arm or leg until you see a doctor to help with the pain.

7. Most fractures heal without surgery and just need a cast without any long-term issues.

8. Your bone will heal even if it feels weak after your cast is first removed. It will eventually become just as strong as the rest of your bones and be no more likely to break.

Types of Broken Bones

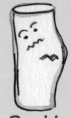

Buckle fracture — *one side of the bone bends, creating a little 'buckle'*

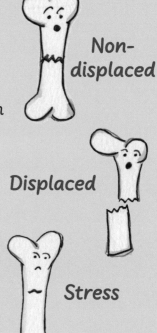

Buckle

Greenstick fracture — *one side of the bone breaks, causing the other side to bend*

Closed fracture — *the bone breaks without hurting the skin*

Non-displaced

Open (compound) fracture — *the bone breaks through the skin*

Non-displaced fracture — *the bone breaks but stays in place*

Displaced fracture — *the bone breaks and no longer lines up; a doctor may need to put the bone back into the right position so that it will heal correctly*

Displaced

Hairline (stress) fracture — *a tiny break in the bone*

Stress

Comminuted fracture — *the bone breaks into more than two pieces or is crushed*

Growth plate fracture — *a break in the growth plate (part of a bone that is still growing)*

Growth plate

Treating Broken Bones

1. Broken bones need rest, rest, and more rest to heal, so they should be moved very little.

2. To help limit movement, you will be placed in a splint or cast. This helps your broken bone to rest and heal, and also helps with pain.

3. You'll need to wear your splint or cast for several weeks to several months. It depends on which bone was broken and where it is located in your body. Your doctor will tell you exactly how long you need to wear it.

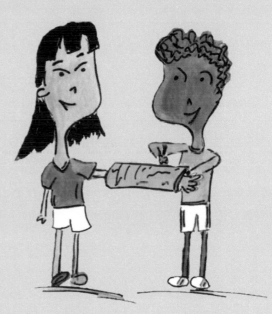

4. Sometimes a broken bone may have moved out of place. This is called a **displaced fracture**. In order for it to heal, a surgeon may move the bone back into the right place. This is called a **reduction**. Sometimes this can be done in the exam room, but other times it has to be done in the operating room, or 'OR'.

Taking Care of Your Cast

1. Keep your cast dry unless it is waterproof! Cover your cast with a plastic bag when taking a bath or shower.

2. Don't put anything into your cast, including powders, lotions, and small toys, even if it itches, because this could cause an infection. Try using cool air from a hairdryer instead.

3. If your cast cracks, let your doctor know! Try to look every day for cracks or tears.

4. If the cast has a sharp edge, you can pad the area to protect your skin.

5. Call a doctor if your cast:
   a. Makes your fingers/toes feel numb
   b. Turns your fingers/toes colors like white or blue
   c. Causes your fingers/toes to have trouble moving
   d. Has a weird smell or drainage
   e. Makes your limb become more swollen
   f. Is causing blisters or cuts
   g. Is causing fevers
   h. Makes your skin turn red or raw

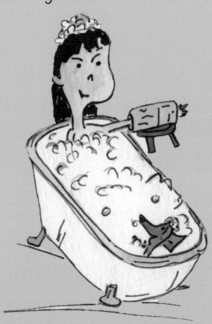

6. Moving with a cast can be tricky, but devices like crutches, walkers, and wheelchairs can help!

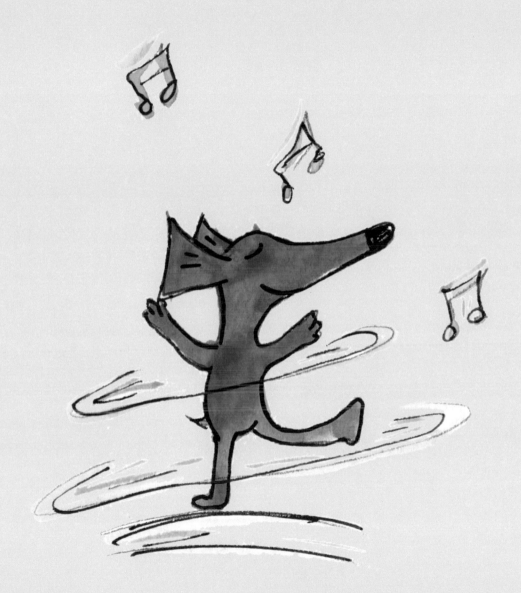

Doctor Words

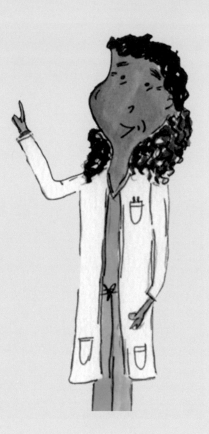

Orthopedic surgeon — a special doctor who takes care of the musculoskeletal system which includes bones, joints, ligaments, tendons, and muscles

Fracture — another name for a broken bone

Sprain — tearing or stretching a ligament

Ligament — a band of tissue that holds two bones together

Joint — where two bones meet (like your knee)

Tendon — a piece of tissue that connects a bone to a piece of muscle

Sedation — medicine that makes you sleepy so a doctor can put your bone back into the right position without hurting you

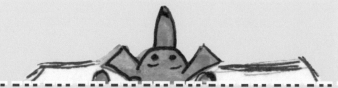

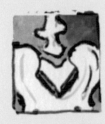

X-ray — a special test that takes pictures of your bones and looks for breaks

Closed reduction — when a doctor moves your broken bone back into the right position. You may be given pain medicines and sedation so you will not feel it.

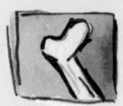

Open reduction — when a doctor moves your broken bone back into the right position in the operating room, or OR for short. You'll be asleep for this and won't feel a thing!

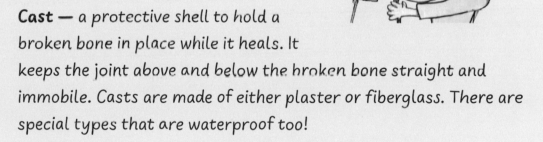

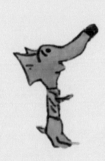

Cast — a protective shell to hold a broken bone in place while it heals. It keeps the joint above and below the broken bone straight and immobile. Casts are made of either plaster or fiberglass. There are special types that are waterproof too!

Splint — similar to a cast but is used when your arm or leg is swollen. It does not go all the way around your arm/leg like a cast. After your swelling improves, you may get your splint replaced with a cast.

Notes

Notes

Meet the Author:
Dr. Maria Baimas-George

Maria Baimas-George MD MPH is a surgeon, training to specialize in abdominal transplantation. Inspired by her patients and mentors, she writes and illustrates books explaining medical and surgical conditions to children and their loved ones. Her goal is to create books that provide useful information to help with understanding and to offer comfort and hope.

WINNER OF THE 2021 SILVER TOUCHSTONE AWARD

Awarded for exceptional performance in patient safety, clinical outcomes, efficiency & service excellence

Please visit us online at
www.StrengthOfMyScars.com to learn more about our team and story and see our full collection of available books.

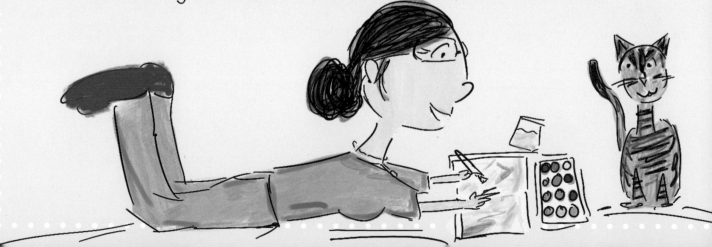